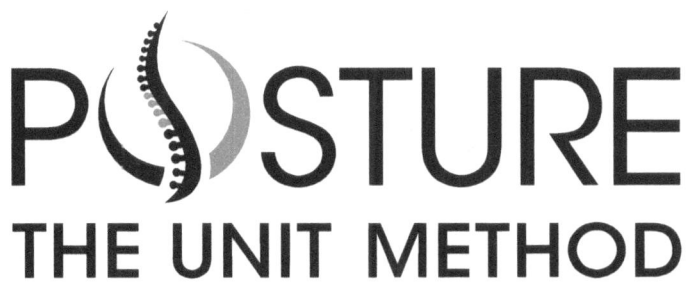

P⟨⟩STURE
THE UNIT METHOD

A New Way for Anyone to Look Great
and Feel Amazing

I0425463

D.B. Heil

CONTENTS

PREFACE

The Unit Method presents a new, self-help approach to posture for daily living. This easy method is for anyone who wants to routinely use their body in a way to reduce or prevent muscle pain, renew health, and enhance appearance. But why offer a new look at posture? The reason is simple: traditional explanations provide an incomplete view of what posture is and does. Posture affects almost every aspect of health—from metabolism to bone density—starting in childhood, so its implications for lifelong health make it a study worth pursuing. The Unit Method proposes a unique interpretation of this remarkable subject, with the belief that understanding posture contributes to the successful practice of it as well as to the enjoyment of its benefits.

In the discussion of posture, circumstances and questions exist that deserve mentioning. Special situations, such as the compromise of the body's structure from misuse, loss of muscle tone, illness, or injury, create distinct challenges. Professional guidance is recommended in these cases. The concept of "good posture" may not be the same for everyone. Also, the length of time it takes for a person to renew the body's structure differs depending on individual circumstances. Practicing posture, for most people, requires perseverance, but ultimately it should feel rewarding and be relaxing.

Seek a professional medical evaluation before applying this or any health resource. Scrutinize all posture resources carefully and at your own risk. It is advised to read these chapters in order. Please find a more complete study of available exercise therapy in the resources. Please read and agree to the complete set of disclaimers that follows.

D. B. Heil

DISCLAIMERS

- Evaluate and practice any posture program under the guidance of a medical professional.
- Do not use posture as a substitute for good nutrition, exercise, or medical care.
- If any exercise causes pain, stop and consult a doctor.
- Avoid correcting another person's posture.
- For a more comprehensive study of posture and posture exercises, see the resources.
- Evaluate and apply this advice and all posture resources at your own risk.

The author assumes no liability regarding undesirable outcomes related to this resource or to the resources provided.

ACKNOWLEDGEMENTS

The author is indebted to the authors cited in the resources and to many others, but especially to Bess Mensendieck who brilliantly merged science with the power of observation to analyze posture.

Genuine appreciation is also due to the libraries and librarians of Michigan who cheerfully and professionally facilitated the research by fulfilling endless requests for titles that led to the development of the Unit Method.

CHAPTER 1

UNDERSTAND POSTURE

Posture's countless benefits are available to anyone.

Posture: A Process for Strength

The Unit Method regards posture not as skeletal alignment, but as *the ability to move, work, and rest according to the body's design for the purpose of creating strength.* When used by design, the body generates strength from childhood to old age. Alignment is one outcome of posture, and the skill of sitting or standing well is only part of the continuous process. The body's organs and tissues receive posture's positive effects, and every body part participates in its application. Posture's potential to boost health is available to anyone who will apply its skills. The power comes through enabling seven other processes that take advantage of gravity while preventing damage from it. In other words, the Unit Method maintains that the ability to use the body according to its design creates strength by enabling the body to continuously accomplish the following processes:

- Align all biological systems to flow with the least amount of stress and compression.

- Harness gravity to stimulate nerve conduction to the entire body.
- Use voluntary muscles to wisely distribute body weight.
- Use voluntary muscles to resist external forces safely.
- Harness gravity to stimulate maximum muscle resistance.
- Harness gravity for building muscle strength and flexibility.
- Harness gravity as a force for easier work and movement.

Expected Results of Posture

- Muscle and bone strength
- Circulatory and digestive system strength
- Maximum oxygen intake and delivery to cells
- Preservation of body shape
- Reduction and prevention of pain
- Production of physical energy
- Increased calorie burn

The Unit Method Vocabulary
The following set of terms assists in applying the Unit Method.

Unit: One of seven specific sections of the body designated as a complete unit of weight.

Alignment: The relative position of any part of human anatomy or unit of body weight.

Neutral: The best position for the entire body and its units during rest or movement. Neutral provides the body its most efficient weight distribution and the best alignment of every part of human anatomy at any time.

Center of gravity (COG): A concentration of weight in the pelvis. The COG acts as a foundation for weight distribution, a point for resisting and distributing gravity, a pivot point for movement, a stabilizing force for balance, and a source of energy for work.

Crown of the head: The highest point on the top of the dome of the cranium.

Ear axis: An invisible horizontal straight line connecting the left and the right ear.

Shoulder axis: An invisible horizontal straight line connecting the shoulder joints.

Hip axis: An invisible horizontal straight line connecting the hip joints.

The Purpose of Units

Units are individual weight masses of the body, visible to the naked eye and useful for the purpose of analyzing the body position from the crown of the head to the toes on the feet. By organizing the body into seven units of weight, posture becomes easy to see. By observing the outline and contours of a fully clothed body, it is possible to analyze the position of the units in relationship to each other. Well-arranged units result in the safe distribution of weight and the best placement of all the body's functioning parts.

The Power of Alignment

The Unit Method maintains that every part of human anatomy has its own alignment, or relative position, and that the body's organs and tissues benefit when functioning in their best position. It is important to note that the skeletal and muscle tissues are uniquely dependent on each other. As a continuous, cooperative alliance, these two systems lose or gain strength together. When muscles in conjunction with the skeleton are aligned according to their design, teams of muscles all over the body share weight bearing, build up muscle mass, and minimize damage. If the body carries weight for long periods of time without efficient skeletal and muscle alignment, the muscles weaken for many reasons. They carry more weight than they are designed to carry, they carry weight in stressful positions for which they are not designed, and some

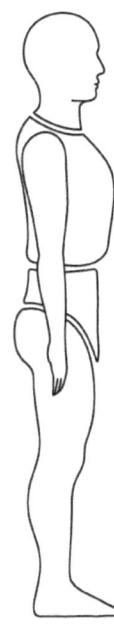

muscles become underdeveloped from lack of use and stiffen up in not-so-normal positions. The practice of posture in daily activity develops muscle strength, starting in childhood. It also helps internal organs stay uncrowded and strong, and it keeps the body's seven units aligned over the course of a lifetime. To discuss the health-giving power of posture, the Unit Method expands the word "alignment" to encompass the needs of the entire body.

The Body's Seven Units
A body unit is made up of its total mass, including its interior systems and contents. The body's seven units and approximate weight of each unit for a 150-pound person are as follows:

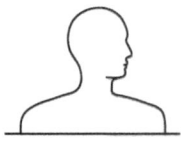

- Crown unit: Head and neck, 18 pounds.
- Cage unit: Upper torso from base of the neck to the waist, 34 pounds.
- Two shoulder units: Left and right arm from shoulder to fingers, 9 pounds each.
- Center of gravity unit: Pelvis region, including pelvic bone and contents, 28 pounds.
- Two hip units: Left and right leg from gluteus to toes, 26 pounds each.

The Force of the Center of Gravity
The center of gravity unit is the foundation for all other units. It holds the COG, the main concentration of weight inside the pelvis area, slightly below the belly button. The COG position affects the shape, movements, and functions of the entire body. The high, centered position is referred to as the neutral COG. A high, stable, and centered COG is a source of energy for work.

A neutral pelvic bone supports the neutral COG. Neutral puts the top horizontal ridge of the pelvic bone directly above the pubic bone, and it keeps this top ridge horizontally straight. The pelvic bone angle can shift out of neutral when the top ridge leans forward or backward, or it can slant diagonally sideways. It is also possible for the right or left side to shift slightly in front of the opposite side. Being out of neutral affects the muscles of the back and hips, and it makes muscles work harder all over the body. Posture and strong muscles hold the pelvic bone and the COG in place. The pelvic bone and COG positions can be detected by observing the body contours.

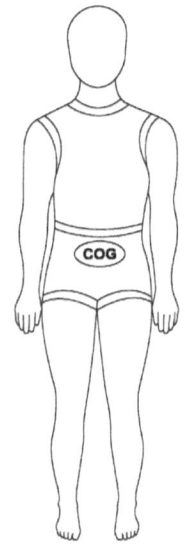

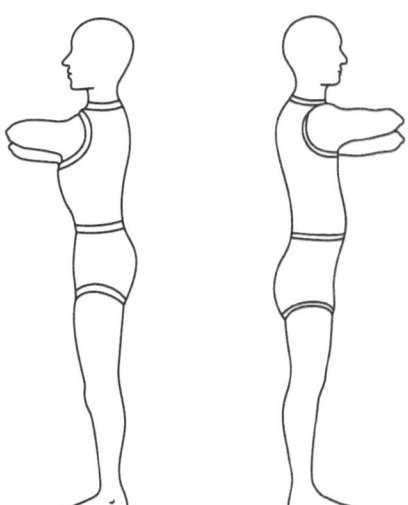

In the following chapters, the Unit Method offers techniques for preserving neutral alignment of the body's units of weight, strengthening the muscles, and improving health through routine activities while taking no time from the day.

CHAPTER 2

STAND AND SIT FOR STRENGTH

After my single hour of exercise ends, my twenty-three hours of exercise begin.

Three Standing Exercises

Three different exercises provide options for learning to stand in neutral. Some people may not be able to reproduce the positions completely. It is not useful to force the body into a tense, painful position. Long-term strength training, careful stretching, and practice help the body regain the ability to generate the neutral stance. The first exercise is brief, the second exercise is detailed, and the third exercise supplies instructions for standing with the body weight distributed on only one leg. The detailed second exercise is followed by comments on the elements of the exercise, and by a quick-reference summary. Breathe, relax, and begin.

Easy Two-Leg Exercise for Strength
Directions
Make a 12" × 12" masking-tape square on the floor.
Stand inside the square.
Keep legs straight and knees very slightly bent.
Make feet and toes point straight ahead, *not* angled in or out.
The balls of the feet will be 1 or 2 inches apart and heels about 3 inches apart.
Let arms hang straight, palms face back.
Rest the bases of thumb joints on side seams of pants or skirt.
Place the head so the ears are above the shoulders.
Look straight ahead.
Gently extend the crown of the head slightly upward.
Breathe deeply.
Imagine you are the president.

Applications

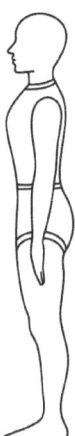

- Standing in line
- After strenuous exercise
- For greetings and handshakes
- While coughing or sneezing
- Going outside on a cold day
- After swinging a golf club
- Putting on makeup
- Talking on the phone

Detailed Two-Leg Exercise
Directions:
Wear form-fitting clothes.
Stand facing a full-length mirror.
Hold a small mirror in one hand.

Front view:
Face the full-length mirror.
Stand up straight, breathe, and relax.
Place feet 2–3 inches apart, and pointing straight ahead.
Make legs straight.
Slightly relax knees; do not hyperextend.
Distribute body weight lightly onto balls of feet.
Feel resistance in ankle and feet muscles.

Side view:
Turn sideways to reflect the body side view in the full-length mirror.
Position feet and legs as above.
Observe the body side view in the full-length mirror by looking in the hand mirror.
Firmly press butt muscles together.
Contract and pull up front abdominal muscles.
Use these muscle contractions to produce a slightly concave low-back curve.
Gently raise rib cage until sternum is high and slightly diagonal.
In upper back, gently position scapulae (shoulder blades) flat against the back.
Make upper-back curve appear slightly convex.
Align shoulder axis directly over hip axis.
Let arms hang straight, palms face back, thumbs touch pant side seams.
Align ear axis directly above shoulder axis.
Form rear outline of neck to a slight concave curve.
Place chin at a 90-degree angle.
Extend crown of the head slightly and gently upward.
Breathe deeply.

Rear view:
Turn the back side of the body to reflect in the full-length mirror.
Observe in the hand mirror.
Check to see if shoulder blades are pressed flat against upper back.
Check to see if shoulder axis and hip axis are horizontal.
Return to front view to recreate the neutral position.
Breathe and relax.

Detailed Two-Leg Standing Observations
Hip Units
When a body stands in neutral, gravity travels a direct path from the crown of the head down through the hip joints, the legs, and finally to the feet. Neutral hips are held symmetrical, the hip axis kept level, and the legs straight. People suffering from hyperextended knees may keep the knees slightly bent. Each foot fully supports weight, but the ball of each foot provides the main point of resistance against the floor. The ball of each foot, including the big toe, presses down, resisting against the force of gravity. This creates muscle resistance in feet and ankles. This resistance against gravity is a feeling of push-back more than it is pushing down. The ball of each foot may be scrunched closer to the heel to lift the arch. The toes scrunch close together.

Standing with angled-out feet should be avoided, except for temporary stability. The overuse of the angled-out feet position contributes to causing the body's center of gravity to sink down and forward, pulling the lower spine into a deep curve and pelvic organs out of neutral. The angled-out position puts stress on hip and leg muscles, rotating them outward. This causes an eventual loss of muscle tone.

Center of Gravity Unit
Observe the position of the COG by looking at the side view of the body's outline. A neutral COG unit and neutral pelvic bone angle are visible when the human head is centered over the horizontal axis connecting the shoulders. Also, the ear axis is lined up directly above the shoulder and hip axes. (Ears are seen above the shoulders.) The chest is high. The angle of the sternum slopes diagonally, and the upper back curve is slightly convex, not hunched. The lower back curve is slightly concave. The abdomen appears flat. The hips are level, and straight legs are close together.

Cage Unit
From a side view, the sternum is high, and it slants slightly diagonally. The upper back curve is slightly convex. Scapulae are pressed flat against the upper back. The back and backbone look mostly smooth. If the backbone looks extremely bumpy, the muscles are out of neutral.

Shoulder Unit and Crown Unit
The crown of the head is the body's highest place. Lifting the crown slightly with a gentle upward stretch decompresses the body. This upward stretch should not cause pain. The head is held centered over the neutral shoulder axis so that the rear outline of the neck forms a slight concave curve. Ears align directly over the shoulders. The chin is at a right angle. This position prevents double chin. Arms hang straight, and palms face back. This position keeps triceps in place to help hold the body upright or to swing back and forth while walking. This prevents flabby triceps. This position gives the shoulder muscle power for its tasks and builds it up. Most people keep continuously twisted or bent arms and curved fingers, resulting in stiff muscles and arms that do not hang straight.

Quick Reference for Two-Leg Standing Exercise
From the side view:

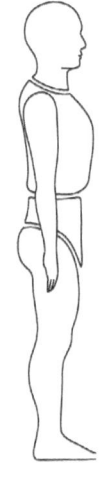

Crown of the head is held high.
Rear curve of the neck is slightly concave.
Chin is at a right angle.
Ear axis is directly above shoulder axis.
Shoulder axis is directly above hip axis.
Sternum is high and diagonally slanted.
Curve of upper back is slightly convex.
Curve of lower back is slightly concave.
Legs are straight.
Knees are not hyperextended.

From the front view:

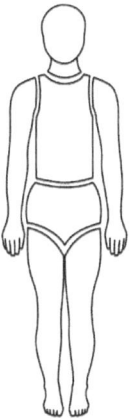

Face looks straight ahead.
Shoulder axis is level.
Hip axis is level.
Arms hang straight.
Palms face back.
Legs are straight and close together.
Feet point straight ahead.
Body weight is distributed evenly over the arches.
Light pressure is distributed on balls of scrunched feet.

Stand for Strength
Single-Leg Standing Exercise

Standing on both legs gives gravity a direct path from the crown of the head through the hips and down to the arches and balls of both feet. Single-leg standing slightly diverts gravity to the arch and ball of just one foot. When the body is in neutral, this single-leg exercise builds muscle strength in the hip units. People who lack balance should hold on to a stable piece of furniture. If single-leg standing occurs often without the body being in neutral, the hip muscles can become weak, leading to developments such as loss of symmetry in the hip axis and a shifting of the neutral COG.

Directions:
Stand in neutral.
Consciously flex muscles of butt and hips.
Keep front part of the right foot on the floor.
Raise the heel of the right foot up about 2 inches off the floor.
Distribute body weight onto the left foot.
Keep hips unmoved.
Hold for a minute.
Lower the right heel back down to the floor.
Distribute body weight to both feet.
Repeat the exercise with the left leg and foot.
Finish by distributing body weight on both feet.

Do:
Spend equal time supporting weight alternately on the right and left foot.
Keep the supporting leg straight.
Prevent the supporting hip from moving out sideways.
Keep symmetry in the hip axis.
If you struggle with balance, put your hand on a straight back chair or counter.

Sit for Strength
Strength training, stretching, and practice help accomplish neutral sitting. Many people need to bring the body back into neutral often, because they are not accustomed to the position. Over time, it feels energizing. It's important to breathe deeply. By sitting in the neutral position, you may find total strangers commenting on how good you look.

Sitting Exercise
Directions:
Sit close to the front edge of a level chair seat.
Place legs close together and parallel.
Place feet flat on the floor side by side.
Point feet straight ahead.
Gently press balls of feet and scrunched toes against the floor to create muscle resistance.
Keep ankles, knees, hips, and chin at 90-degree angles.
Rest arms on the thighs or on a table, with a bend at the elbow and palms facing down.
(If seated on a low stool, let arms hang straight and palms face back.)
Place head so ears align above shoulders and shoulders align above hips.
Raise the crown of the head gently up to the ceiling to decompress the upper body.
Breathe deeply, smile, and look around.
Imagine you are a queen.

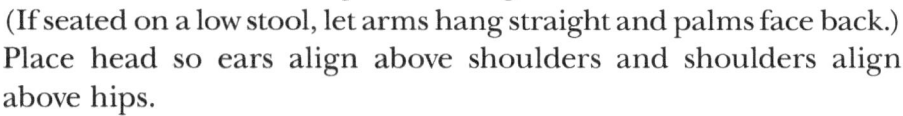

Note: Scoot farther back into a chair and rest against the back of the seat if your head and neck can be supported in the neutral position.

Sit Down on a Chair Exercise
Directions:
Stand with your back side to a chair seat.
Put straight legs close together, feet pointing straight.
Touch the seat's edge with the back of your legs.
Slide the foot of one leg slightly back under the chair.
Tighten gluteus and abdominal muscles.
To sit, descend by shifting supported body weight from front leg onto the under-the-seat leg.

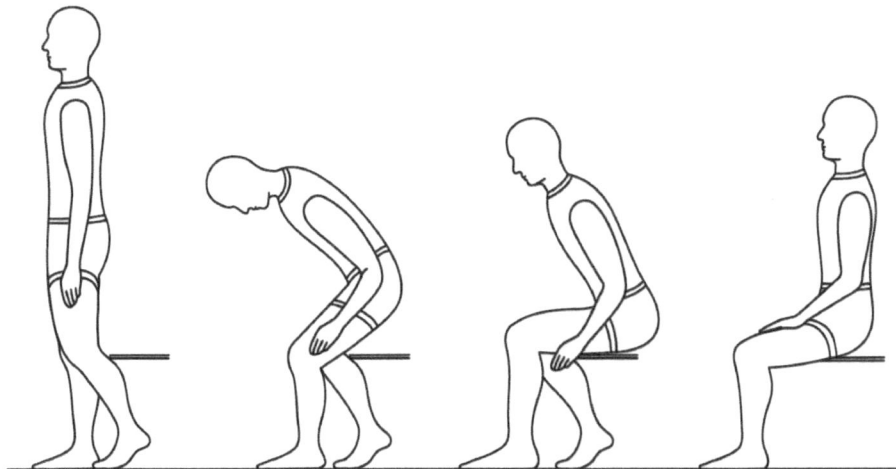

Keep the COG neutral, and lean upper body slightly forward as you slowly transfer body weight onto the seat.
Sit with a tall crown in the neutral position.
Slide the rear foot forward to rest beside the other one.

Rise from a Chair Exercise
Directions:
Scoot your weight close to the chair seat's front edge.
Place legs close together, feet pointing straight.
Slide one foot slightly back under the chair.
Flex gluteus muscles and abdominals, and lean upper body slightly forward.
To rise, contract gluteus muscles to help scoop up and propel the COG forward and up.
Smoothly shift supported body weight from the under-the-seat leg to the forward leg.
Stand up straight.
Slide the under-the-seat foot forward so it is next to the other foot.
Distribute body weight evenly on both legs.

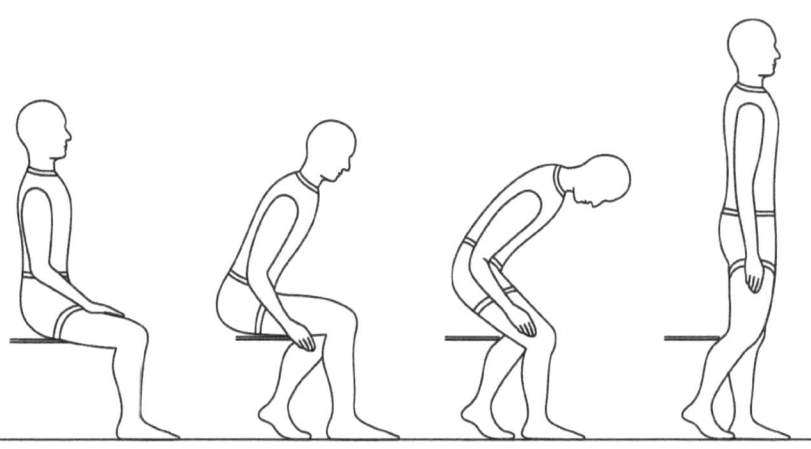

Do:
Keep the neutral angle of the pelvic bone unchanged.
Move with controlled movements.
Allow legs to do most of the work, not arms.
As you sit down, exhale, and then inhale when you are seated.
As you rise exhale, and then inhale when you are standing.

Exercise for Neck Strength
This exercise completes the standing or sitting exercises. It strengthens neck muscles, helps prevent double chin, and lessens compression on the neck and upper body.

Directions:
Sit on a chair or stand in neutral.
If possible, observe the body in a mirror.
Breathe deeply in and out to relax.
Imagine a royal crown is suspended immediately above your head. Gently, slowly, slightly extend your head upward until it fits perfectly into the crown.
Breathe again, and slowly release the muscle contractions.

Do:
Look straight ahead.
Place your chin at a right angle to your neck.
Make the upward movement slight.
Be gentle.

Don't:
Overdo it.

Car Seat Exercise for Strong Neck Muscles
Sit in a car seat and situate the crown unit so it is high and centered over the shoulder axis. The ears should be in position above the shoulders, not forward. Use pillows if needed to reshape the seat position. Adjust the seat and head rest for support if applicable.

Move in and out of a Midsize Car Seat for Strength
To move the body into a small or midsize car seat:
First, place the COG on the seat.
Swing both legs in together.
Scoot farther back in the seat.
Sit in neutral.
To get out of a small or midsize car seat:
Swing both legs out of the car together.
Scoot the COG close to the edge of the seat.
Keep feet pointing straight.
Stagger your feet by placing one foot about three inches ahead of the other.
Scoop the body out and up, supported by both legs.
Stand up in neutral.

Bow the Head Forward Exercise
Directions:
Sit in neutral.

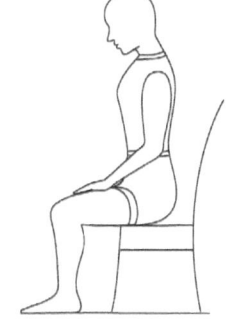

Bow the head slightly forward.
Curve only the neck forward.
Keep the entire back in neutral.
Return the head completely to neutral.
Breathe deeply.

The bowed head exercise helps to develop strength in the trapezius muscle, and preserve its flexibility and neutral shape. Do not hold the bowed position for long periods. Remaining too long with a bowed head causes a loss of muscle strength. People who pray, read, study, craft, play instruments, or use electronics will benefit from strength training exercises for strong neck and back muscles.

Find a Chair that Produces Muscle Strength
A firm, flat seat creates a neutral angle for the pelvic bone and produces core muscle resistance in the neutral position. If a chair is very soft or overstuffed, try sitting on the front edge of the seat. To recline in stuffed chairs, office chairs, and car seats, use pillows to restructure the chair's shape in order to support the neutral body position. The back of a reclining chair should be high enough to fully support the head without pushing it forward. An ottoman should be slightly lower than the seat of a chair to save knees from hyperextension. If a chair is paired with a desk, table, or counter, the levels of the seat and table top should coordinate to prevent hunching over.

Make Adjustments to Exercise Equipment Chairs
Adjust the seats on exercise machines to support neutral positions. Some equipment, especially recumbent bike seats, have slanted back rests with no head support. This puts the head and neck at an awkward forward position and stresses the trapezius muscle. When possible, adjust slanted exercise equipment seats so

the entire body is aligned in neutral. Add a pillow to support the back and neck when needed.

Sitting on the Floor Exercise

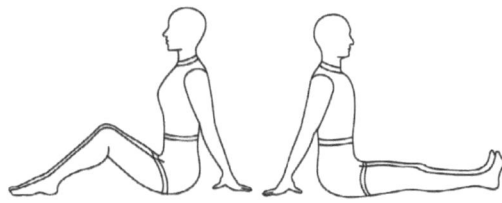

Hold the upper body in neutral with a high crown of the head. Place legs symmetrically, straight or bent. Avoid sitting in the "lotus" position. It twists ankles, and it compresses blood vessels and nerves.

For sitting with crossed legs, do not place a leg or ankle to rest upon the other one. Instead, position one bent leg slightly ahead of the other; the sides of both feet and legs resting on the floor. This prevents leg compression and keeps ankles from turning inward.

To get up and down from the floor, let legs do the work. Using a controlled lunge with good form develops leg and hip strength. If balance is a problem, support the body with hands placed on a table or walking stick. Keep a high crown. Start and finish with neutral standing.

CHAPTER 3

WALK BY DESIGN

The pursuit of stronger muscles produces stronger brains, hearts, and metabolisms.

Walking Exercise

This method, which applies to basic walking, preserves energy and uses the position of the COG for added power. The COG leans or slightly falls forward. (For advice on Nordic walking, fitness walking, and treadmill workouts, see the resources.) If the body is viewed from above, the right shoulder moves slightly forward, and at the same time, the left hip moves forward, and vice versa. The COG is the pivot point for the body's left-side/right-side pivoting movements. Large muscles in the pelvis help to swing the legs. The steps are small to keep each foot from landing too far ahead of the COG. Weight on each foot is distributed from the firm heel strike straight through to the ball of the foot and big toe for the push-off.

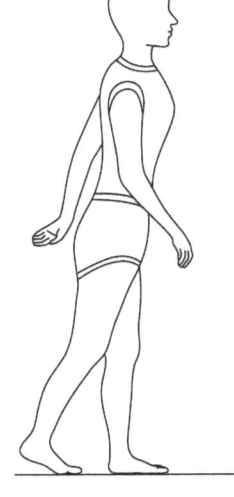

Beginning position:
Stand tall in neutral.
Place ears directly over the shoulders.
Look straight ahead.
Make palms face back.
Make feet point straight ahead.

The movement:
Lean the entire neutral body very slightly diagonally forward.
Swing the right shoulder and arm forward.
Simultaneously swing the left hip and leg forward.
Walk and continue to alternate the movements.
Take small steps.
Step down with a firm heel strike.
Land on each heel, and push off with each big toe.

Do:
Swing arms equal distance, straight forward and straight back.
Feel the forward swing of each shoulder and arm help propel the body forward.
Feel each leg swing forward from the hip.
Look straight ahead.
Walk confidently with a firm step.

Don't:
Look down.
Lean forward at the hips.
Swing the arms diagonally back and forth.

Please note:
If the walking exercise is difficult to achieve due to previous changes in the body structure, you can keep walking. Pursue small, gradual improvements. Adding daily strength training

exercises is encouraged. Do not force the body into a position that is uncomfortable.

Push a Cart for Strength

This method of pushing and walking behind a cart builds core muscle strength.

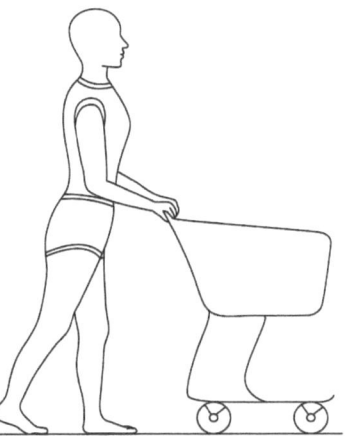

Directions:

Stand in neutral.
Raise the crown of the head high.
Press upper arms in close against the body.
Hold the cart close to the body with both hands.
Firmly hold the cart handle.
To push, incline the entire body slightly diagonally forward.
Take small steps forward.
Feel the entire body pushing the cart.

Don't:

Curve the upper body over the cart handle or lean forward at the hips.

Push a Wheelchair and Preserve Strength

To push someone in a wheelchair, adjust the handles to match the proportions of your body. Stand up straight. Do not hunch over. Install bicycle handlebar extenders if the handles are too low.

Improve Feet Strength

Strong feet muscles develop by applying natural weight distribution patterns for movement throughout the day, and by taking advantage of the stationary neutral foot position. Strength training and flexibility exercises for the hips and legs will also improve feet strength. It is advantageous to avoid feet underuse or overuse.

Stationary Neutral Foot Position Exercise
Directions:
Stand in neutral.
Keep legs side by side and parallel.
Make feet point straight ahead.
Keep the space between the balls of the feet 1 or 2 inches.
The distance between the heels is 2–3 inches.
Scrunch toes close together.
Let little toes barely touch the ground.
Feel balls of the feet and big toes press slightly down. (This pressing down is a feeling of resistance or push-back against the floor.)
Keep ankles at 90 degrees.
Feel slight muscle resistance in feet and ankle muscles.

Shoes that Develop Feet Strength
Invest in shoes that allow the feet to move naturally according to their design. Shoes should have some cushioning, a flexible sole, arch support, and a low heel. Shoes and socks should fit. Flip flops and high heels are among shoes that do not allow natural movement; their use should be limited. The Unit Method does not recommend wearing shoes with negative heels.

CHAPTER 4
WAYS TO BUILD STRENGTH DAILY

The practice of posture allows every system of the human body to function without stress.

Go up and down Steps to Build Strength
Going up Steps Exercise
Directions:
Approach the bottom step.
Face the steps and stand in neutral.
Lean the entire neutral body forward at a slight diagonal incline.
Step up to lift the body weight with each alternating leg.
At the top of the stairs, stand up completely straight.

Do:
Feel like the upper body glides up smoothly on an invisible slide.
Keep a hand lightly on the rail.

Keep feet pointing straight ahead and legs close together.
Keep spine and neck motionless.
Keep chest high.
Lean the COG slightly forward with each step.
Let leg and gluteus muscles do the work.
Straighten each leg as it steps up.

Don't:
Pull the body weight up by hands on the rail.
Move your neck back and forth.
Lean at the hips.
Hunch your back.

Going down Steps Exercise
Directions:
Slowly approach the top step.
Pause and stand in neutral.

Observe the dimensions of the steps.
Put a hand on the rail.
Lower the first foot and leg and then alternate
to descend.

Do:
Feel as if the weight of the butt glides smoothly
down an invisible slide.
Keep a hand on the rail.
Keep feet pointing straight ahead.
Keep upper body straight and crown high.
Let leg and gluteus muscles do the work.

Lean the Upper Body Forward Exercise
This movement strengthens back muscles and improves their flexibility. It should not be held for long periods of time. It is useful for

tasks such as bending forward over a sink or drinking fountain. The upper body leans forward above the waist. The lower front abdominal wall stays vertical. The COG and pelvic bone remain unmoved in the neutral position. The back muscles receive a safe stretch.

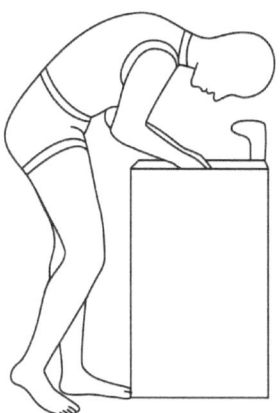

Directions:
Stand in neutral, close to and facing a counter, table, or bed.
Distribute most body weight onto the front part of the feet.
Bend the knees slightly.
Tighten abdominals in front.
In the rear, press gluteus muscles together and down.
Press tail bone firmly into the body.
Lean over above the waist only (above the belly button).
Return to the upright neutral position and relax.

Do:
Feel like the lower abdominal muscle is a fence or wall as high as the belly button.
Feel the upper body bend forward over the imaginary wall.
Feel the tail bone as an anchor for a gentle stretch of the lower back muscles.
Keep legs straight or slightly bent at the knees.
Feel weight distributed on the front part of the feet.
Feel muscle resistance in the front of the ankles.
Breathe out on the way forward.
Pause and breathe in.
Breathe out on the way back up.
Pause and breathe in again.
Return to a neutral stance.

Don't:
Hold the forward position for a long period of time.
Hyperextend the knees.

Strength from Reaching a Low Object
Movements such as loading or unloading the clothes dryer can strengthen the leg muscles. Squats, lunges, and kneeling movements are all safe and acceptable. The upper body remains in neutral. Bending forward from the hip can be done safely, but this movement is not recommended for lifting a heavy object.

To reach for a low object and lift it, first kneel down, then draw the object to the body and hold it close to the COG. Use the legs to lift the body weight back to a standing position. For a wider base of stability during this task, try placing one leg slightly in front of the other, or temporarily rotate legs and feet outward to stand up, and then return feet to the neutral position.

Put On and Take Off a Jacket Exercise
Directions:
Stand in neutral.
Hold a light jacket or sweater.
Keep your back and neck perfectly still.
Use the movement of the arms to put on the jacket and to remove it.

Do:
Practice this exercise in front of a mirror.
Hold your head high.
When finished, let arms hang straight and palms face back.
Breathe deeply.

Eat and Drink for Shoulder, Arm, and Neck Strength
Sit in neutral at the dinner table. Use the muscles of the shoulder to bring food or drink to the mouth. Hold the neck almost

motionless and the crown high. Occasionally bend the crown and neck forward if needed, or lean forward from the hips. Always return the upper body to neutral. These techniques will also strengthen the ability to swallow.

Easy Arm Muscle Flexibility Exercise
Most people spend countless hours with bent arms. Consequently, muscles in the front of the arms lock up in a shortened position, and as a result, the arms no longer hang straight. The following stretch helps restore the muscles' original length and flexibility. This easy exercise may be done for short periods at any time of day.

Directions:
Sit on a chair without arm rests, or stand in neutral.
Allow both arms to hang straight.
Make palms face back.

Strength from Cutting in the Kitchen
The following method is for cutting food such as raw squash. It takes stress off small muscles of the wrist, and it strengthens shoulder and core muscles. It preserves the neutral shape of the upper back. The technique harnesses the force of gravity by using the weight of the COG. If the table or counter top is at waist level or slightly lower, then the stable upper body weight and COG contribute to the task.

Be careful. Use care and common sense when cutting with any sharp tool.
Directions:
Place the food item to be cut on a cutting board at waist level or slightly lower.
Stand in neutral.
Press arms in close to your sides.

Position shoulders down.

Bend elbows at about a 90-degree angle.

Hold the food carefully with one hand.

To cut, increase pressure on the knife in your other hand by moving your stabilized body weight back and forth.

Do not move arms too far away from the COG.

Hold wrists firm and straight as possible.

Keep the head held high.

Feel the weight of the stabilized upper body and COG contribute to the work.

Vacuum to Build Up Hip Muscles

This method takes stress off smaller muscles of the arms, and it exercises hip muscles and abdominals.

Directions:

Stand next to the vacuum cleaner.

Press upper arms in close to the sides of your body.

Grasp the vacuum cleaner handle.

Step forward to push.

Keep the vacuum as close as possible to the body.

Let legs support and move the body back and forth.

Try not to extend the arms too far out from the body.

Try not to lean forward from the hips.

To pull, step back to return to the original standing position.

Keep the head consistently high.

Pick up an Object on a Table Exercise
Directions:

Stand in neutral.

Stand directly in front of and close to a small object on a table.

Reach for the object with both hands.

Keep a high crown.

Exhale and draw the object close to the COG.

Lift and carry the object close to the COG, and breathe normally.

(To lift an object from, or lower an object to the floor, hold the object close to the COG, and then use your legs to move the body up and down in the neutral position.)

Carry a Purse for Strong Shoulders
Stand in neutral and keep the horizontal shoulder axis level and directly above the hip axis. Occasionally alternate carrying a purse or bag on different shoulders. If possible, with your arm hold the bag close to the body. Hold a very heavy bag with both hands, centered and close to the COG. Avoid carrying a bag that causes the shoulders to slant, or the head to move forward.

Use Electronics to Preserve Strength
Sit or stand in neutral to use cell phones, computers, and electronic devices. If necessary, prop up small devices on a table at an angle to avoid having to hunch over. Adjust the distance and height of a desk computer to your proportions and wear prescription computer glasses. Strengthen and stretch the appropriate muscles with exercise, including neck, back, shoulders, and hands. Add alternative movements and stretches to repetitious work. Change positions when possible, and take breaks.

More Ways to Pursue Muscle Strength through Posture

- Buy furniture that supports neutral positions.
- Hang wall mirrors at eye level.
- Provide comfortable child-sized furniture for young children.
- Provide extra pillows to support children when they sit.

- When children study at a table, provide angled study boards to prop up study materials. (A pillow or stack of books works for this.)
- Use angled study boards for yourself.
- Avoid studying and watching TV in bed.
- Set up computer stations to promote neutral positions.
- Put computers at eye level.
- Use an adjustable office chair.
- Use a stand-up desk.
- Mount a mirror beside a desk to view your head and neck position.
- Invest in prescription eyeglasses for computer work.
- Use neutral positions with all electronics.
- Learn stretches and strength exercises to do at home, work, school, and for travel.
- Practice strength training exercises in front of a mirror.

CHAPTER 5

TECHNIQUES TO KEEP
THE COG NEUTRAL

There is no reason for the pursuit of strong muscles to stay in the domain of athletes.

Develop Symmetrical Strength

Body symmetry helps keep the COG in its best position: high, stable, and centered. Related groups of muscles on the body's left and right side can lose symmetry and become mismatched in many ways. The muscles can develop differences in strength, flexibility, size, and positional symmetry. Habitual movements, repetitious work, uneven weight bearing, injury, and illness all contribute to a loss of symmetry in the muscles and in the shape of the left and right side of the body. In addition, a person's dominant side may become stronger than the nondominant side, and the dominant side muscles can become tired and contracted. Posture and strength training support or restore body symmetry.

Techniques to keep symmetry:

- Use symmetrical posture positions for work and weight bearing.
- Use both hands to push a cart, close a drawer, or put away groceries.
- Use the nondominant arm to open doors, wash dishes, or brush teeth.
- Alternate shoulders to carry a bag.
- Swing both legs together to get out of bed or a chair.
- Do core exercises.
- Strengthen the body's nondominant side with exercise.

Do not attempt any unsafe movement that compromises safety.

Breathe Sideways to Keep the COG Centered
The Unit Method cautions against belly breathing, or pushing the stomach forward and out to inhale. This practice forces the center of gravity down and forward. When the COG is pushed forward, it takes organs and the spine along with it, weakening the diaphragm and abdominals. In addition, breathing by moving the shoulders up and down contributes to neck pain and TMJ. In order to preserve the neutral body shape and build diaphragm strength, the diaphragm should expand mostly to the sides. The shoulders remain level, and front abdominals stay fairly flat. Although the lungs and diaphragm expand outward to some degree in all directions, expansion mostly to the sides helps preserve strength.

Inhalation
Breathe in through the nose. This sends clean oxygen and a gas called nitric oxide (NO) to the cells. The body makes NO, a neurotransmitter, in the nasal passages using certain nutrients. NO

helps dilate blood vessels and improves everything from heart disease to growing hair. It is also used in the process of building and repairing muscles.

Exhalation
Breath out through the mouth. Exhaling removes cell waste. It prevents the blood from becoming acidic and the blood vessels from constricting due to excess carbon dioxide. Exhaling may contribute to fat loss. Fat is oxidized as H_2O and CO_2, molecules that leave the body by exhalation.

Breathing Exercise
Directions:
Stand and face a mirror to observe the body.
Place the palm of one hand flat on the abdomen just below the belly button.
Smile and breathe in deeply by expanding lungs out, mostly to the sides.
Try to keep the flat hand from going forward.
To breathe out, open your mouth as if to laugh.
Breathe out deeply.
Keep the head and shoulders from moving up and down.
Repeat the exercise several times.

Lifted-Diaphragm Breathing for Strength Training
During both phases of resistance exercise, it is possible keep the diaphragm up by exhaling in order to minimize gravity's downward force on the COG. Exhaling flexes the abdominal muscles, and helps hold the COG in neutral. Resisting with the diaphragm up reduces downward pressure on the internal organs and the core muscles. It may help weight lifters prevent hemorrhoids. This is the pattern: exhale during the concentric contraction, pause briefly to breathe in, then breathe out on the eccentric

contraction, pause and breathe in again. Complete all repetitions with this pattern, using an even rhythm. Remember to inhale and exhale fully.

Lifted-diaphragm breathing with biceps curls exercise:
Stand and hold free weights in neutral starting position for biceps curls.
Exhale slowly while lifting the weights toward the shoulders.
Pause and inhale slowly.
Exhale while lowering the weights back to starting position.
Pause and inhale slowly.
Repeat this pattern.
Keep a slow, even rhythm.

Muscles that Keep the COG High
The development of strong abdominals, glutei, and pelvic floor muscles with exercise will help maintain the high, neutral COG. Pelvic tilt exercises and pelvic floor muscle strengtheners, including the Kegel, should be added to any strength training plan for men or women. Some therapists recommend pelvic floor muscle exercises to improve health situations specific to men. For exercise options, see the resources. *Some people should not attempt Kegel exercises. Professional medical advice is strongly advised.*

Develop Flexible Muscle Strength
Flexibility is a specific type of muscle strength that assists in supporting the COG and the entire body posture. Flexible strength includes the muscles' ability to extend and move in all the ways associated with the muscles' design. In addition to this, a flexible muscle has the ability to support, work, bend, lengthen, and then pull back to the neutral starting position and relax without pain. For most people, flexibility must be developed and maintained by posture, resistance exercise, and stretching.

Flexibility provides many practical results. It counteracts a muscle's tendency to remain contracted after injury, hard work, repetitive positions, and periods of inactivity. It facilitates blood flow and maintains the normal cooperation of muscles all over the body by preventing muscles from locking up in a shortened position. It heals pain. It improves posture.

Flexibility exercise can be learned from a professional physical therapist or trainer. Any exercise done with bad form may alter the shape of the body or do other damage. Overstretching can be harmful as well. Few flexibility trainers are educated in all types of stretching, and mistakes in form exist in some exercise books and resources. The Unit Method recommends engaging in personal research for training options, and exercising with the guidance of a well-trained therapist.

See the resources for further study. Evaluate all therapies carefully and consult a medical professional before starting a stretching program.

RESOURCES

The following resources do not represent an endorsement. Evaluate all resources carefully and at your own risk.

Posture Books

Egoscue, Pete, with Roger Gittines. *Pain Free: A Revolutionary Method for Stopping Chronic Pain*. New York: Bantam, 2000.

Gokhale, Esther, with Susan Adams. *8 Steps to a Pain-Free Back: Natural Solutions for Pain in the Back, Neck, Shoulder, Hip, Knee, and Foot*. Stanford, CA: Pendo, 2008.

Harvey, Jean-Francois. *Cure Back Pain: 80 Personalized Easy Exercises for Spinal Training to Improve Posture, Eliminate Tension, & Reduce Stress*. Toronto: Robert Rose, 2016.

Lagerwerff, Ellen, and Karen A. Perlroth. *Mensendieck Your Posture and Your Pains*. Garden City, NY: Anchor/Doubleday, 1973.

Manocchia, Pat. *Anatomy of Exercise: A Trainer's Inside Guide to Your Workout*. Buffalo, NY: Firefly, 2009.

Meeks, Sara. *Walk Tall: An Exercise Program for the Prevention and Treatment of Osteoporosis*. Gainesville, FL: Triad, 1999.

Mensendieck, Bess. *Look Better, Feel Better*. New York: Harper, 1954.

Novak, Janice. *Posture, Get It Straight! Look Ten Years Younger, Ten Pounds Thinner, & Feel Better Than Ever!* Andover, MN: Expert, 2006.

Strength Training Books

Anderson, Bob, Bill Pearl, Ed Burke, Jeff Galloway, and Jean Anderson, Illustrator. *Getting Back in Shape: 32 Workout Programs for Lifelong Fitness*. Bolinas, CA: Shelter, 2006.

Brill, Peggy, and Gerald Secor Couzens. *The Core Program: Fifteen Minutes a Day That Can Change Your Life*. New York: Bantam, 2003.

Fekete, Michael. *Strength Training for Seniors: How to Rewind Your Biological Clock*. Alameda, CA: Hunter House, 2006.

Gonzalez-Wallace, Michael. *Super Body, Super Brain: The Workout That Does It All*. San Francisco: HarperOne, 2011.

O'Driscoll, Erin. *The Complete Book of Isometrics: The Anywhere, Anytime Fitness Plan*. Hobart, NY: Hatherleigh, 2005.

Pagano, Joan. *Strength Training for Women: Tone Up, Burn Calories, Stay Strong*. New York: DK, 2013.

Rogers, Phyllis. *Over 40 and Gettin' Stronger: An Easy-to-Learn Strength Training Workout for Adults*. Marietta, GA: Fitness Press, 2004.

Schlosberg, Suzanne, and Liz Neporent. *Fitness for Dummies*. Hoboken, NJ: Wiley, 2010.

Flexibility Books

Anderson, Bob, and Jean Anderson, Illustrator. *Stretching: 20th Anniversary; Revised Edition.* Bolinas, CA: Shelter, 2000.

Anderson, Bob, and Jean Anderson, Illustrator. *Stretching in the Office.* Bolinas, CA: Shelter, 2002.

Chabut, LaReine, with Madeleine Lewis. *Stretching for Dummies.* Hoboken, NJ: Wiley, 2007.

Esmonde-White, Miranda. *Aging Backwards: Reverse the Aging Process and Look 10 Years Younger in 30 Minutes a Day; Updated and Revised Edition.* New York: Harper Wave, 2018.

Esmonde-White, Miranda. *Classical Stretch: The Esmonde Technique; The Textbook.* San Francisco, CA: Pearson, 2006.

Knopf, Karl. *Foam Roller Workbook: Illustrated Step-by-Step Guide to Stretching, Strengthening & Rehabilitative Techniques.* Berkeley, CA: Ulysses, 2011.

Knopf, Karl. *Stretching for 50+: A Customized Program for Increasing Flexibility, Avoiding Injury, and Enjoying an Active Lifestyle.* Berkeley, CA: Ulysses, 2005.

Martin, Suzanne. *Stretching, the Stress-free Way to Stay Supple, Keep Fit, and Exercise Safely.* New York: DK, 2005.

McAtee, Robert. *Facilitated Stretching: 4th Edition with Online Video.* Champaign, IL: Human Kinetics, 1999.

Roberts, Melanie, and Stephanie Kaiser. *Idiot's Guides: Stretching.* New York: Alpha, 2003.

Wharton, Jim and Phil. *The Wharton's Stretch Book: Featuring the Breakthrough Method of Active-Isolated Stretching.* New York: Three Rivers, 1996.

Specific Therapy and Exercise Books

Bowman, Katy. *Simple Steps to Foot Pain Relief: The New Science of Healthy Feet.* Dallas, TX: BenBella, 2016.

Brin, Lindsay. *How to Exercise When You're Expecting for the 9 Months of Pregnancy and the 5 It Takes to Get Your Best Body Back.* New York: Plume, 2011.

Butler, Sharon J. *Conquering Carpal Tunnel Syndrome and Other Repetitive Strain Injuries: A Self-Care Program.* Oakland, CA: New Harbinger, 1996.

Chabut, LaReine. *Lose That Baby Fat! Bouncing Back the First Year After Having a Baby: A Mom Friendly Fitness Program.* New York: Evans, 2006.

Davies, Clair. *The Frozen Shoulder Workbook: Trigger Point Therapy for Overcoming Pain & Regaining Range of Motion.* Oakland, CA: New Harbinger, 2006.

Davies, Clair. *The Trigger Point Therapy Workbook Third Edition: Your Self-Treatment Guide for Pain Relief.* Oakland, CA: New Harbinger, 2013.

Diamond, Janet, and Zipora Schulz, Illustrator. *Exercises for Airplanes and Other Confined Spaces.* New York: Excalibur, 1996.

Hlavac, Harry F. *The Foot Book: Advice for Athletes.* Mountain View, Ca: World, 1997.

Huey, Lynda, and Robert L. Klapper. *Heal Your Hips: How to Prevent Hip Surgery and What to Do If You Need It*. Nashville, TN: Turner, 2015.

Huey, Lynda, and Robert L. Klapper. *Heal Your Knees: How to Prevent Surgery and What to Do If You Need It; Revised and Updated Edition*. Lanham, MD: Evans, 2007.

Johnson, Joan. *The Healing Art of Sports Massage: A masseuse to dozens of sports superstars shows you how to: Prevent injury, Improve performance, Relieve sore, stiff muscles, Speed recovery, Reduce stress, and more...* Hampton, NH: Mindstir Media, 2012.

McIlwain, Harris H., Debra Fulgrum Bruce, Joel C. Silverfield, Michael C. Burnette, and Bernard F. Germain. *Winning with Back Pain: Leading Specialists Show You How to Beat Back Pain and Take Control of Your Life*. New York: Wiley, 1997.

Morrone, Lisa. *Overcoming Back and Neck Pain: A Proven Program for Recovery and Prevention*. Eugene, OR: Harvest House, 2008.

Neporent, Liz. *Fitness Walking for Dummies*. Foster City, CA: IDG Books, 2000.

Pascarelli, Emil. *Dr. Pascarelli's Complete Guide to Repetitive Strain Injury: What You Need to Know about RSI and Carpal Tunnel Syndrome*. Hoboken, NJ: Wiley, 2004.

Peterson, Cynthia. *The TMJ Healing Plan: Ten Steps to Relieving Headaches, Neck Pain, and Jaw Disorders*. Alameda, CA: Hunter House, 2010.

Prudden, Bonnie. *Pain Erasure the Bonnie Prudden Way*. Lanham, MD: Evans, 2002.

Schlosberg, Suzanne. *Fitness for Travelers: The Ultimate Workout Guide for the Road.* Boston, MA: Houghton Mifflin, 2002.

Sobel, Dava, and Arthur C. Klein. *Arthritis, What Exercises Work: Breakthrough Relief for the Rest of Your Life, Even After Drugs and Surgery Have Failed.* New York: St. Martin's, 2015.

Stein, Amy. *Heal Pelvic Pain: A Proven Stretching, Strengthening and Nutrition Program for Relieving Pain, Incontinence, IBS, and Other Symptoms without Surgery.* New York: McGraw-Hill, 2009.

Struna, Monika. *Self-Massage: Touch Techniques to Relax, Soothe and Stimulate Your Body.* London: Vermillion, 1994.

Walter, Claire. *Nordic Walking: The Complete Guide to Health, Fitness, and Fun.* New York: Hatherleigh, 2009.